Cut Your Prescription Drug Costs

*The Resource You Need
To Start Saving Now*

Cynthia Mauck, CPhT

ISBN-13: 978-1480084025

Cover design by Jennifer Rose

Cover photo by Cynthia Mauck

Dedicated to.....

My mother Virginia Hall for her loving support through the years.

The sheer joy of reading to your children led me to a love of words and, far down the

road, this book.

Thanks Mom!

ACKNOWLEDGEMENTS

Thanks to the following people for you support and help.

Shana Adkins, RPh. Shana is a pharmacist with whom I work. She reviewed several chapters in which the information needed to come from someone with a degree in pharmacology − namely Generics; Splitting Pills; Buying in Bulk. Thank you for your helpful suggestions and knowledgeable input.

Jennifer Rose for your cover design. Reed Coleman for your generous spirit. My mother Virginia Hall for your helpful suggestions. Roxanne Hunter for providing me with some great information. Linda Barr Batdorf for your help with the back cover text.

ABOUT ME

I've worked as a pharmacy technician for over 7 years. I'm nationally certified and am licensed to practice in the state in which I live and work. Prior to this career, I worked 25 years in news media — mostly in television news. I have a B.A. in Journalism. It's time to follow through on my intention when I left television — to use my skills to help people.

INTRODUCTION

My phone rings in the mail order pharmacy where I work. A customer is calling in reply to a message a pharmacy technician left about the high cost of one her medications. I have the unenviable task of informing her that the co-pay is $443.28 for a 90-day supply. Once she has recovered from the shock she says "you're kidding me" (a common response). Dejectedly she says "this is medication I have to have, there is no way I can afford this. I guess I'll have to talk to my doctor or else stop eating".

Sadly, I'm limited in the time I have to deal with customers. As much as I would love to pass along all the cost cutting measures I know, I simply haven't the time. Usually I will mention one or two ways to cut; beyond that I can't be the help I'd like to be. I'm writing this book so I can give that help. Not only to my pharmacy's customers but everyone who currently takes, or will be taking medication.

This book can help those with insurance, and those without it. I won't promise every saving measure can be applied to all of your drugs. With life comes change. As we grow older we are likely to be taking more and more medications. Some of the savings measures may be used in your future.

DISCLAIMER

Nowhere in this book am I advising which medications to use, which pharmacy to patronize, or which cost-cutting measure to take. Actual drug names are used as examples only. The true costs of medications are used, but no customer, plan or insurance company names are given.

Always consult your doctor and/or a pharmacist before making any changes to your medication. Your good health is more valuable than money in the bank.

CONTENTS

Chapter 5

Chapter 6

Chapter 7

Chapter 8

Chapter 9

Chapter 10

1

Take Stock

Get information from your insurance company

It's time for action. Boning up on the provisions of your prescription drug plan will prove invaluable, so start with calling your insurance company. You need to know what you are paying right now for each of your medications. There are other things you need to know that will affect your efforts to bring down costs. For instance, coverage for one drug might be completely denied. Another might incur an ancillary fee. A medication your insurance has covered for years might now require a prior authorization or step therapy. This might be the first time you have a deductible to pay. Knowing all this will help greatly in your decision-making.

To make this process easy for you, I've provided:

- A section to write the name of your insurance company, its customer service phone number, and your member ID number.
- A form to list all your medications and their costs for a 30-day supply at retail and a 90-day supply through mail order.
- The questions to ask.
- A page to make your own notes.

Have the book open to these pages when you call, and write the information in the spaces provided.

First, it will help to acquaint yourself with terms that will be used now and in later chapters.

Ancillary Fee—what you pay if you take a brand drug when a generic equivalent is available. You pay the cost of the generic PLUS the cost of the difference in price between the generic and the brand drug. Not all insurance companies charge ancillary fees. If yours does, that's a reason to consider taking a generic drug.

Co-pay—the amount you pay for the cost of a drug. Your insurance pays the rest.

Day Supply—the number of days for which the prescription is filled.

Dose—how much of that medication you take each day.

Drug Form—how the medication is packaged: in a tablet, capsule, bottle, vial, inhaler, etc.

Formulary—sometimes called a preferred drug list. This lists the medications your insurance company covers, and usually will indicate which co-pay tier each drug falls into.

Prior Authorization—Sometimes your insurance company will not let you take a drug until documentation is submitted by your doctor to the insurance company. The documentation they need from the doctor is proof that you've taken at least one or two other medications for that condition and they weren't effective. If you have taken other medications and they weren't effective, there is a good chance the prior authorization will be granted. Getting a prior authorization can take a while, so it's something worth asking about when you call your insurance company.

Retail—local pharmacy.

Step Therapy—This is similar to a prior authorization. In this case, your insurance company requires you to try one or two medications in the same drug class before they will allow you to fill the drug that requires step therapy.

Insurance Company Name _____

Phone Number _____

My Insurance ID Number _____

DRUG STRENGTH FORM	DOSE	30-DAY COST	90-DAY COST

Now it's time to call your insurance company and ask:

Please send me two copies of my formulary.

What are the co-pay tiers for my plan and what is the co-pay for each tier?

Generic _____   Brand Formulary _____   Non-Formulary _____

What is the maximum day supply for retail? _____

What is the maximum day supply for mail order? _____

Do any of my medications require a prior authorization?

Yes ___   No ___

If yes, then what medication is preferred?

_____

Do any of my medications require step therapy?   Yes ___   No ___

If yes, then what medication(s) is/are preferred?

_____

Do I pay ancillary fees?   Yes ___   No ___

       If yes, what will be the total cost? $_____

Do I have a deductible to pay?   Yes ___ No ___

       If yes, how much? $_____

Does the deductible apply only to the account holder?

       Yes ___ No ___

Does the deductible apply to all my medications, or only those in the top tiers (the brand names)?   All ___   Top tier ___

Can I use coupons or co-pay assist cards?   Yes ___   No ___

NOTES

2

Generics

Your Single Greatest Savings Source

What is a Generic Drug?

Basically, a generic is the same chemical from a different manufacturing company.

The Food and Drug Administration's (FDA) definition:

"A drug product that is comparable to a brand/reference listed drug product in dosage form, strength, route of administration, quality and performance characteristic, and intended use."

Huh?

Let me restate this in a nongovernmental way.

- A generic drug contains the same active ingredient as its brand name.
- If the brand name comes in tablet form, capsule form, ointment form, etc., so will its generic.
- The generic is available in the same strengths as the brand drug.
- Route of administration? The generic is taken the same way as the brand: by mouth, via injection, apply to the skin, etc.
- Quality and performance characteristic? The generic medication works in the body like the brand name does. It is absorbed and used by the body just as the brand name is.
- The generic and brand treat the same medical condition.

A generic drug looks different than its brand. It will have different markings on every single tablet for different manufacturers and strengths. Look on the prescription bottle's label to see what is being dispensed. If you're concerned you aren't receiving the correct medication, call a pharmacist to verify what the drug is.

Savings

No doubt you know that generic drugs cost considerably less than brand name drugs. Here is an actual example of the savings:

A customer called me to renew one of her medications that recently became available as a generic. Her co-pay when she last ordered the brand name medication was $100.00 for a 90-day supply. When I placed the order, I watched as the electronically-submitted claim came back from her insurance company. She was thrilled to hear the co-pay was now $10.00. She is saving **$360 a year** on one medication. How is that for an incentive to switch to a generic?

"Generics Don't Work For Me"

In dealing with customers, I occasionally hear some people say they can't take generics, claiming they have "never worked for me" or "I had a nasty reaction to the generic."

Perhaps some people have an aversion to trying a generic drug simply because the word generic conjures up images of something inferior. During my teen years, a warehouse supermarket opened in our town. That store carried some generics of brand name foods. It was the first time I had seen soup cans that didn't have a recognizable label with a well-known company name on them. The generic soup was packaged in a laughably plain manner, with only black printing on a white label. The packaging was so unappealing that I had a negative view of anything generic for a long time.

Consider this. A generic drug has been around for a long time. When a drug is first released to the public the pharmaceutical company that developed it, gets a patent for "approximately 12 years" per the FDA. Sometimes that patent can be extended for another three to five years. Once it expires, other pharmaceutical companies can produce it and sell it. The competition drives the price down. At this point, the drug has been on the market long enough to have weathered the test of time and proven its safety and effectiveness.

If you are more interested about the effectiveness of generics, watch these interviews with doctors when Lipitor went generic in November 2011:

abcnews.go.com/Health/video/brand-drugs-generics-15050710
    www.youtube.com/watch?v=u_yVXgXm2L8

How Changes to Your Insurance Plan Can Bust Your Budget

You may have reasonably low co-pays for your brand drugs. Let's say $25.00 for a 30-day supply at retail and $50.00 for a 90-day supply through mail order. Those prices are typical. One insurance plan handled by my pharmacy had the following 90-day mail order co-pays in 2011 for its members:

Generic - $10.00
Formulary Brand Name - $50.00
Non-Formulary Brand Name - $100.00

The year 2012 saw those costs change dramatically. And I do mean dramatically. Those members now have four co-pay tiers. All of those co-pays are now a percentage of the total contractual costs of the drugs.

Lowest-cost Generics — 5%
Other Generics — 10%
Formulary Brand Name and High Cost Generics — 30% + $100 yearly deductible
Non-formulary Brand Name — 50% + $100 yearly deductible

Due to that change, some generic co-pays dropped to as little as $0.29, with other generics costing more than the 2011 set co-pay of $10.00 for all generics.

Co-pays for the brands have generally gone up. For example, in 2011 a customer paid $50.00 for 90 capsules of a medication for attention deficit disorder. In 2012, his cost was $130.33 (30% of the contractual cost). That's a whopping 160% increase. Earlier in 2012, he paid *more* than $130.33 for that medication because his yearly deductible was applied to his co-pay.

This can happen to you. If it's not rising premiums, it's your co-pay for a doctor visit or your prescription medications. The plan change listed above is a good example of how insurance companies are overtly pushing you toward generics. Would a 5% or 10% co-pay on a generic drug and no deductible entice you to take generics if you aren't already?

If your prescription plan moves from set co-pays to percentage co-pays, call your insurance company before you order a refill of an existing prescription or start on a new medication. A customer service representative will be able to tell you your cost.

"Don't I Have to Take What My Doctor Prescribes?"

Yes and no. Yes, you take the medication. No, you don't have to take the brand if you want the generic. If the generic is what you want, ask your doctor to write for that. If you feel uncomfortable asking, try what I said to my doctor. When I found my bad cholesterol level was sky high, I simply asked, "If it's ok with you, I'd like to try a generic first." She said "I already had Simvastatin in mind for you." I've been fortunate that other doctors I've seen over the years asked *me* if it was ok for them to prescribe a generic. Absolutely. Yes indeed. I wouldn't have it any other way.

I suggest you contact your insurance company and ask for copies of the formulary for your plan. Get two copies - one for you and one to give your doctor. It will help you both know which drugs will be lower cost for you. If you have internet access, you can probably find it at your insurance company's website. It might be called a preferred drug list, rather than a formulary.

Am I Taking A Generic?

If you are unsure if your medications(s) are generic, call a pharmacist, or visit:

www.drugdigest.org

The site was created by Express Scripts, Inc., one of the largest mail order pharmacies in the U.S. It's a great site aimed at the general public. Search by drug name to find a lot of useful information about the drug. You'll be able to see if the drug is available as a generic or not. In many instances, you can see color photos of your medication along with the names of the companies that manufacture it. You can also read what medical condition the drug treats, its possible side effects, how to store it, when to call your doctor about side effects, etc. It's a very resourceful site which includes a money saving tool worth checking out.

When Will My Medication Go Generic?

If you'd like to know when a drug is scheduled to go generic, check this list.

DRUG	MONTH/YEAR
Abilify	*April 2015*
AcipHex	*November 2013*
Actonel	*June 2014*
Actoplus Met	*December 2012*
Adcirca	*November 2017*
Advate	*February 2019*
Advicor	*September 2013*
Aggrenox	*July 2015*
Aloxi	*October 2015*
Alphagan P	*January 2022*
Ampyra	*January 2026*
AndroGel	*August 2015*
Asacol	*January 2014*
Atacand	*December 2012*
Atacand HCT	*December 2012*
Avelox	*February 2014*
Avodart	*May 2015*
Avonex Administration Pack	*September 2026*

Azor	*October 2016*
BeneFIX	*April 2019*
Benicar	*October 2016*
Benicar HCT	*October 2016*
Betaseron	*September 2026*
Boniva	*May 2023*
Byetta	*July 2020*
Bystolic	*April 2020*
Cancidas	*September 2017*
Celebrex	*May 2014*
Cerezyme	*August 2013*
Chantix	*November 2020*
Cialis	*May 2018*
Cimzia	*February 2024*
Cipro HC	*January 2015*
Combivent	*December 2015*
Copaxone	*November 2014*
Coreg CR	*December 2015*
Crestor	*July 2016*
Crixivan	*August 2021*
Cymbalta	*December 2013*

Detrol	*September 2012*
Detrol LA	*May 2020*
Dexilant	*June 2020*
Differin	*March 2023*
Diovan	*September 2012*
Diovan HCT	*September 2012*
Enablex	*June 2016*
Enbrel	*February 2014*
Epogen	*May 2015*
Epzicom tablets	*March 2016*
Evista	*March 2014*
Evoxac	*December 2012*
Exelon Patch	*January 2019*
Exforge	*December 2017*
Exjade	*April 2019*
Focalin XR	*June 2016*
Follistim - vial	*January 2018*
Follistim – cartridge	*August 2019*
Fosamax PlusD	*June 2013*
Fuzeon	*December 2015*
Gilenya	*February 2019*

Gleevec   *July 2015*

Hepsera   *March 2015*
Humira   *December 2016*

Intuniv

                                           September 2015
Janumet   *October 2026*
Januvia

                                           October 2026
Kaletra - tablet   *December 2016*
Kaletra - oral solution   *November 2020*
Kuvan   *November 2025*

Letairis   *July 2018*
Lialda   *June 2020*
Lidoderm   *November 2012*
Loestrin24 Fe7   *January 2014*
Lovaza   *March 2015*
Lumigan   *August 2014*
Lunesta   *May 2014*

Lupron	*December 2016*
Lupron 3.75 mg	*May 2014*
Lyrica	*June 2019*
Maxalt	*December 2012*
Maxalt-MLT	*December 2012*
Micardis	*January 2014*
Micardis HCT	*January 2014*
Namenda – oral solution	*April 2015*
Namenda - tablets	*January 2015*
Nasonex	*July 2014*
Neulasta	*October 2015*
Nexavar	*January 2020*
Nexium	*May 2014*
Niaspan	*September 2013*
Nitrostat	*September 2018*
Norvir - tablet	*December 2016*
Norvir - solution	*January 2015*
NuvaRing	*October 2018*
Opana ER	*January 2013*
Oracea	*April 2022*

Orencia	*October 2019*
Ortho Evra	*May 2016*
Ortho Tri-Cyclen Lo	*December 2015*
Oxytrol	*April 2015*
Pataday	*December 2015*
Patanol	*December 2015*
Pegasys	*November 2019*
Proair HFA	*September 2023*
Procrit	*May 2015*
Pulmozyme	*July 2015*
Rapamune	*January 2014*
Rebif	*September 2026*
Relpax	*June 2017*
Remicade	*September 2018*
Renagel	*September 2014*
Renvela	*March 2015*
Revatio	*September 2012*
Revlimid	*October 2019*
Reyataz	*June 2019*
Rilutek	*June 2013*
Rituxan	*September 2016*

Sandostatin	*January 2017*
Sensipar	*September 2018*
Seroquel XR	*November 2016*
Simponi	*March 2026*
Solodyn ER	*August 2018*
Spectracef	*October 2016*
Spiriva	*March 2027*
Stelara	*September 2023*
Strattera	*May 2017*
Sustiva	*March 2015*
Sutent	*August 2021*
Synagis	*October 2015*

Tamiflu	*June 2017*
Tarceva	*November 2018*
Tarka	*February 2015*
Tazorac gel	*June 2014*
Tekturna	*January 2019*
Tekturna HCT	*January 2019*
Temodar6	*August 2013*
Teveten	*December 2015*
Thalomid	*December 2023*
TOBI	*October 2014*
Travatan	*June 2015*
Travatan Z	*June 2015*

Trilipix	*January 2014*
Truvada	*September 2021*
Tykerb	*September 2020*
Tyvaso	*November 2018*

Valcyte	*March 2013*
Velcade	*May 2017*
Vesicare	*May 2019*
Viagra	*April 2020*
Victoza	*August 2022*
Vigamox	*March 2020*
Viracept	*April 2014*
Viread	*January 2018*
Vivelle-DOT	*December 2013*
Vytorin	*April 2017*
Vyvanse	*June 2023*

| WelChol | *June 2015* |

Xeloda	*June 2014*
Xolair	*December 2018*
Xyrem	*June 2024*

Zetia	*December 2016*
Zometa	*March 2013*
Zomig	*May 2013*
Zomig spray	*May 2021*
Zytiga	*December 2019*
Zyvox	*May 2015*

3

Mail Order

Saves Money, Time, and Gas — a Win-Win-Win Situation

You've switched to generics. You've taken stock of your medications and know the provisions of your prescription insurance plan. When calling your insurance company to get prices, perhaps you noticed that a 90-day supply cost more than a 30-day supply. That's no surprise. But did you do the math and realize by getting a 90-day supply, you one get one month free? Whether your medications are brand or generic, you will lop 33% off your entire bill. This is getting better and better, isn't it?

Mail order has other advantages:
- Save gas (no more driving to a pharmacy).
- Save time (no more standing in line at a local pharmacy).
- Free shipping.
- Orders mailed directly to you.
- You can refill your medications online, via automated phone systems, by calling customer service, or mailing in refill slips.
- You can refill your prescriptions three weeks before you are scheduled to run out of your medication. Some insurance companies allow you to fill a month in advance.
- Medications requiring refrigeration can be purchased through mail order. They are shipped overnight in cold packs.

Most insurance plans allow you to fill your medications through mail order. In fact, some insist you get your maintenance medications through mail order. Those that do usually require that you start filling a prescription via mail order after you've filled it twice at a local pharmacy within a set period of time (usually 1 year).

It's important to note that mail order is not intended for medications you need to start taking immediately or will be taking for a short time. Mail order is intended for maintenance medications — drugs you are, or will be, taking for a long time. When you start taking a drug, it's common for your doctor to prescribe only a 30-day supply. After those 30 days she'll want to run a test to see if the medication is working. If it isn't, she'll either change the medication or change the strength and write another 30-day prescription. The time to make the switch to a 90-day supply is when the doctor finds the strength and dose that works.

My entire pharmacy technician experience has been working for mail order pharmacies. I will walk you through getting started, and help make it work smoothly for you.

My Mail Order Pharmacy _____

Customer Service Phone _____

Customer Service Hours _____

Mailing Address _____

_____

_____

QUESTIONS TO ASK WHEN YOU CALL TO SET UP A MAIL ORDER ACCOUNT

When can I refill my prescriptions?_____

How do I order a refill?

_____

_____

_____

_____

Do I pay up front, or can I be billed?

_____

Can I be set up for automatic refills?   Yes ____   No ____

Can you send bottles with easy opening caps?

      Yes ____   No ____

What is your method of shipping?   (first class, 4th class, UPS, etc)

_____

How long before I get my first order? _____

What is your website? _____

Step 1. Call your insurance company to get the name and phone number of the mail order pharmacy you will use.

Step 2. Call the mail order pharmacy and have them set you up in their computer system. This should only take a few minutes. Have your insurance information handy and a credit card, debit card, or FSA/Health Savings Account card. Some pharmacies will want payment at the time they ship an order, others will bill.

Step 3. Get your prescriptions to the mail order pharmacy. This can be done several ways: you mail them; your doctor phones or faxes them to the pharmacy; ask the mail order pharmacy to transfer them from another pharmacy. A few mail order pharmacies won't transfer in prescriptions from other pharmacies, so ask them if they will or will not do transfers. If you are having your doctor write new prescriptions, ask the doctor to prescribe for 90-days with three refills.

NOTES

NOTES

Making Mail Order Work for You
Let me guide you through how it can work smoothly for you.

Mail in Prescriptions
Even though you can have your doctor phone or fax your prescriptions, it's better if you mail them in. There are two reasons for this.

1. If your doctor faxes a prescription, you won't know if what he wrote was correct until you receive the medication. If the doctor goofs, you'll be stuck with that medication. State Board of Pharmacy laws forbid the return of medications, even if you never open the package or the bottles. Also, your co-pay will not be refunded. Pharmacies won't swallow the cost if the mistake is the doctor's. I've seen customers stuck with some large co-pays because their doctor made a mistake. You can avoid that. ***Look at the prescription before you leave the doctor's office.*** The directions for use are written in a Latin-based shorthand, so have the doctor tell you what that is. Once the correct prescription is in your possession, mail it to the pharmacy. By law, you cannot fax a prescription.

2. Faxes don't always get to the pharmacy. Many times, I've heard customers swear their doctor's office faxed, it, yet we didn't receive it; this is because the doctor's office, in fact, didn't send it. Or they do fax or send it through their computer, but doesn't make it to the pharmacy. I have no other way to explain it than some prescriptions are lost in cyberspace.

Special note about faxing: doctors cannot fax or call in prescriptions for schedule 2 controlled substances.

Definition of a controlled substance—Any drug or therapeutic agent commonly understood to include narcotics, with a potential for abuse or addiction, which is held under strict governmental control, as delineated by the Comprehensive Drug Abuse Prevention & Control Act passed in 1970.

Schedule 2 controlled substances are primarily narcotics and stimulants. These drugs are strictly regulated by the Drug Enforcement Agency (DEA).

Schedule 2 drugs:
- Must be mailed in. The hard copy of the prescription must be mailed, and it must have the doctor's handwritten signature on it.
- Can be prescribed for a 90-day supply, unless the state you live in restricts that (a few do).
- Cannot be refilled. You will need a new prescription each time you need it filled.

Refills
With most mail order pharmacies, you can place a refill order:

- By calling customer service and have a representative place the order.
- Through the internet.
- Through the pharmacy's automated phone service.
- By mailing in refill slips that will come with your orders.
- With automatic refill − if the pharmacy offers that option.

Once you've established mail order service, you'll need to know when and how to order a refill. The earliest most insurance companies allow a refill of a 90-day supply of a medication is 21 days before you are scheduled to run out of your medication. The easy way to figure this out is: find the fill date on the label on your bottle, add 90-days to that date, and then subtract 21 days from that date. This is the earliest you can refill your medication. I recommend doing the refill then. Although it doesn't happen often, I've seen the U.S. Postal service misroute mail all over the country.

Reasons to refill as early as allowed:

- If your prescription is expired or out of refills and your mail order pharmacy will fax your doctor for a new prescription, it takes time to get that done. Some doctors are slow in returning a request. Also, it's not uncommon the request will be denied, because you doctor will want to see you first for labs or an appointment.
- Your medication might be on back order. This doesn't happen often, but sometimes there are manufacturer back orders.
- If your insurance company changes the status of the medication – it now needs a Prior Authorization or Step Therapy – the mail order pharmacy won't be able to fill it until the prior authorization is approved or the step therapy has been completed.

- **Note:** insurance issues can keep you from getting your medication in a timely manner, whether you are getting the medication at retail or mail order.

If you procrastinate and don't order a refill until you have only a few pills remaining and you'll run out of medication before an order can reach you, there are two options:

1. Don't place the order with the mail order pharmacy. Have a local pharmacist call to transfer the prescription(s) to his pharmacy. You can get the medication that day.

2. Call your doctor's office to see if you can get samples. If so, go ahead and order the mail order refill, then get the samples at your doctor's office.

Read Your Mail

It's not uncommon for insurance companies to make changes to plans between the yearly sign up times. If one or more of those changes will affect you, they will send you a letter. For example: one insurance company recently sent letters to some of its customer advising them that their high cost generics were moving to a higher co-pay tier. In those letters, they advised customers what alternative medications they could take to avoid the impending higher co-pays. It literally pays to read your mail.

4

Low, Low, Low-Cost Generics

No Insurance Required!

Now that you know what your insurance co-pays are, it's time to determine if any of your medications can be purchased for less through a retail pharmacy offering low-cost generics.

Does buying a 30-day supply for $4.00 or a 90-day supply for $10.00 beat your insurance co-pays? If so, read on.

I'm making this easy for you. I've provided a list of pharmacies that offer these bargain prices. In addition to the pharmacies offering $4.00 and $10.00 generics, I list pharmacies offering similar programs, but at different prices. Note that some pharmacies charge either a one-time fee or annual membership fees. Read through all of them, as you'll see some pharmacies are *giving away* certain drugs.

The Basics

- You do not use insurance. You pay the pharmacy $4.00 or $10.00 and that's it. No insurance company is billed.

- You do have to give the pharmacy a prescription written by your doctor, nurse practitioner, etc. If you've been filling a medication at another pharmacy and want to transfer it to the pharmacy offering low-cost generics, ask the pharmacy to call the pharmacy where your prescription resides to have it transferred.

Purchasing a 90-day supply is a better deal, but perhaps your doctor only prescribed a 30-day supply. If your doctor wrote at least two refills on the prescription, ask the pharmacist to use those two refills and make it a 90-day supply.

Pharmacies That Offer Low-Cost Generics Programs

Note: some of these pharmacies offer a few antibiotics and diabetic medications for free; one gives free Lisinopril; another gives free prenatal vitamins and children's prescription vitamins.

If you don't have internet access to see each stores generic list, then call and ask if your generics on are their list. If you happen to be in one of the stores, then swing by the pharmacy area. More than likely, the printed list will be available for you to take home.

The pharmacies are listed primarily by lowest to highest cost.

KROGER and its stores that have pharmacies

- **City Market**
- **Dillons**
- **Fred Meyer**
- **Frys**
- **Gerbes**
- **King Sooper**
- **QFC**
- **Ralphs**
- **Smiths**

www.kroger.com/generic/Pages/alpha_listing.aspx

Costs: $4.00 for 30-day supply $10.00 for a 90-day supply

Membership Fee: None

TARGET

http://sites.target.com/site/en/spot/page.jsp?title=pharmacy_generic_drugs_alphabetical

Costs: $4.00 for a 30-day supply $10.00 for a 90-day supply

Membership Fee: None

WALMART

www.walmart.com/cp/1078664

Costs: $4.00 for a 30-day supply $10.00 for a 90-day supply

Membership Fee: None

SHOPRITE – CT, DE, MD, NJ, NY

www.shoprite.com/cnt/Pharmacy.html

Costs: $3.99 for a 30-day supply $9.99 for a 90-day supply

Free: children's prescription multi-vitamins, up to a 30-day supply

Free: prenatal vitamins, up to a 30-day supply

Free: some antibiotics, up to a 14 day supply

Free: some diabetic medications, up to a 30-day supply

Membership Fee: None

HY-VEE – IA, IL, KS, MN, MO, NE, SD, WI

www.hy-vee.com/health/pharmacy/generics/default.aspx

Costs: $4.00 for a 30-day supply $10.00 for a 90-day supply

Membership Fee: None

GIANT EAGLE – MD, OH, PA, WV

www.gianteagle.com/pharmacy/unbeatable-discount-
program#$4/$10GenericsProgram

Costs: $4.00 for a 30-day supply $10.00 for a 90-day supply

Free: Some Antibiotics and Diabetic Medications

Membership Fee: None

GIANT FOOD STORES – MD, PA, VA, WV

www.giantfoodstores.com/shareddev/sharedcontent/SP/SavingsList09/?CFID=4226
7676&CFTOKEN=28013128&jsessionid=8430867b92afb21724da6462f4c32776136
5

Costs: $4.00 for a 30-day supply $10.00 for a 90-day supply

Free: Some antibiotics, up to a 14 day supply

Membership Fee: None

WEGMANS – MD, MA, NJ, NY, PA, VA

www.wegmans.com/webapp/wcs/stores/servlet/CategoryDisplay?storeId=10052&identifier=CATEGORY_513

Costs: $4.00 for a 30-day supply $10.00 for a 90-day supply

Free: some antibiotics

Membership Fee: None

H.E.B. – TX

www.heb.com/pharmacy/rx-rewards.jsp

Costs: $5.00 for a 30-day supply $9.99 for a 90-day supply

Free: Prenatal vitamin

Membership Fee: One time only fee of $5.00 that covers everyone in the family

STOP & SHOP – CT, MA, NJ, NY, RI

www.stopandshop.com/shop_online/pharmacy/generic.htm

Cost: $9.99 up to a 90-day supply

Membership fee: none

RITE AID

www.riteaid.com/pharmacy/rx_savings.jsf

Costs: $9.99 for a 30-day supply $15.99 for a 90-day supply

Membership Fee: None

KMART

www.kmart.com/shc/s/dap_10151_10104_DAP_Kmart+Pharmacy+Savings+Club

Costs: $5.00 for a 30-day supply $10.00 for a 90-day supply

Membership fee: Annual $10.00 enrollment fee for individuals and $10.00 for households. When you join, the $10.00 fee will be added to the price of your first prescription.

WALGREENS

The medications are classified by payment tiers.
www.walgreens.com/pharmacy/psc/psc_overview_page.jsp?ban=rxh_psc_6
Tier 1 - $5.00 for a 30-day supply $10.00 for a 90-day supply
Tier 2 - $10.00 for a 30-day supply $20.00 for a 90-day supply
Tier 3 - $15.00 for a 30-day supply $30.00 for a 90-day supply
Membership Fee: An individual pays a yearly fee of $20.00 to join, $35.00 a year for a family.

CVS

www.cvs.com/promo/promoLandingTemplate.jsp?promoLandingId=healthsavingspass
Cost: $11.99 for a 90-day supply (they don't offer a 30-day supply)
Membership fee: $15.00 annually per person. To cancel, you have to write CVS a letter.

PUBLIX PHARMACY – AL, FL, GA, SC, TN

www.publix.com/pharmacy/Free-Medications.do
Publix does not have a generics program, but does offer a few medications for free.
Free: Lisinopril - Maximum of a 30-day supply (up to 60 tablets). Lisinopril-HCTZ combination products excluded.
Free: some Antiobiotics, up to a 14-day supply

Free: Metformin, up to a 30-day supply (90 tablets) of generic immediate-release metformin (500mg, 850mg, and 1000mg)

5

Split Your Tablets

Take another half off

You take generic mediations. You get one month free by purchasing 90-day supplies of your maintenance drugs through mail order. You might think you can't possibly lower your costs anymore. Yet in some cases, you can slash your costs by 50%.

Before I explain how to do this, I want to stress you should always consult first with a pharmacist and then with your physician.

Here's how this works. Let's say you take one tablet a day of Simvastatin 20mg. Your cost for 90 tablets is a set, generic co-pay of $10.00. If you have your doctor write Simvastatin 40mg, quantity 90, you'll still pay $10.00. But you will get 180 tablets of 20mg by splitting the 40mg tablets in half. You are still taking the 20mg strength your doctor wants you to take, but you are getting 180 days for $10.00 instead of a 90-day supply for $10.00.

Simvastatin 20mg, 90 tablets = $10.00

Simvastatin 40mg, 90 tablets split in half = 20mg, 180 tablets = $10.00

A huge savings? No. It's a $20.00 a year savings. But if you can split more medications, you'll experience greater savings.

Think what you'll save if you split a costly brand name drug. Perhaps it's the only drug that works for you. You've tried the generic of that drug and you had a bad reaction. You've tried other drugs in the same class of drugs, or a similar class of drugs, and only the expensive brand drug works for you. If it's a medication that a pharmacist says you can split and is available in double the strength, then call your doctor for a new prescription for the double strength.

Before splitting pills, make certain your doctor plans to have you on this medication for at least six months. Also, buy a pill splitter. They are inexpensive. I purchased one in 2012 for $4.19. Pill splitters can be found in the pharmacy area of a store. Splitters are easy to use and will come with instructions.

I've used my pill splitter on both of my medications that come in a tablet form. One tablet is scored (has a line across the middle), the other is not. The splitter makes a very clean, even cut with both medications. I push the lid down with a quick motion that takes very little effort.

I will reiterate, not all tablets are meant to be split and never split capsules. Capsules are rarely designed for splitting. Most capsules have a fine, loose powder inside. Splitting one creates a mess and leads to inaccurate dosing. In addition, sometimes the outer shell on tablets or capsules is part of the medication delivery system. For example, special coatings are used to slow down or delay the release of medication. Splitting would stop this delay.

Before splitting tablets, call a pharmacist to see if the drug can be split and if it comes in the strength you will need to split. If so, let your doctor know you want to split your medication and see if he will write a prescription for the higher strength.

6

Buying In Bulk

Buy a lot for very little

You might be able to save money on your least expensive generics by purchasing six months to a year's supply at a time.

Here is a real case scenario.

One of our customers lives in a county that does not fluoridate the drinking water. So her children take chewable fluoride, an inexpensive medication. Fortunately for her, she once worked in a dental office and knows it comes packaged in 1,000 count bottles. She also knows the chewable fluoride costs little.

Cash price for 90 tablets: $10.95
Cash price for 365 tablets: $20.23

If she had continued purchasing 90 at a time, she would have paid $43.80 for a year. By purchasing a year at a time she saved over 50%.

Before you buy in bulk:

- Be certain you will be taking the medication for the length of time you will be purchasing. Make certain the pharmacist fills the prescription with medication that won't expire for a year or more.

- If you are insured, you won't be able to bill your insurance. Insurance companies won't allow a fill of more than a 30- to 34-day supply at retail or 90- to 100-day supply through mail order. So you will be paying the entire cost out of pocket.

- Call several pharmacies to ascertain the lowest cash price before deciding where to buy.
- Since most medications will cost less through your insurance, not many drugs will be cheaper in bulk. To know if purchasing in bulk will work for you, call your pharmacy for pricing.

The list of generics available for $4.00 and $10.00 would be a good place to look. The drugs on those lists tend to be the least expensive drugs.

Think how you much you will save by purchasing in bulk and splitting tablets! Check first with a pharmacist on splitting and ask if the medication will be effective for such a long period.

COUPONS

Anywhere from a little to a lot off your costs

How much you save on one prescription by using a coupon card can vary drastically. Three examples:

1. Recently a customer used two coupons on an order he placed. His co-pay for one drug was $687.00 for a 90-day supply. The coupon took off $600.00. The other coupon took $200.00 off his co-pay for the other medication. On that order alone, he saved $800.00

2. A customer used a coupon that gave him three free months of his medication. The terms of the coupon limited him to a one-month supply each time. Considering the price of his one-month supply was almost $7,000.00 (yes, there are drugs that are that expensive), he was getting quite a bargain.

3. A customer called with a coupon that took only $15.00 off her co-pay for one of her medications. After the other two examples, this may not seem like much, but many coupons are good for up to 12 fills in a year. $15.00 X 12 = $180.00.

Now, to bring you back down to earth, most coupons don't provide the savings seen in the first two examples. But if the brand drug you are taking has no generic available and no similar drug has worked for you, then a coupon can provide financial relief.

What you should know about manufacturer coupons

- Every manufacturer coupon I found stated: Not valid for prescriptions covered or paid for by Medicare (including true out-of-pocket expenses under Medicare Part D), Medicaid, or any other federal or state healthcare programs, such as state pharmaceutical assistance programs.

- Coupons can be called many things: Co-pay assist card, rebate card, savings card, savings program.
- Some websites require you to register in order to receive the coupon. The registration is free and you won't be asked for a credit card. In some cases, these sites offer many other types of support: links to support groups or organizations that will help you with your medical condition; list useful information about the medication; provide phone support with a nurse or specially trained representative; free kits you can order.
- Some coupons need to be activated before using them.
- Manufacturer coupons are meant to be used in conjunction with your insurance.
- Some coupons are 30-day free trials only.
- Not all coupons are meant to be used for 90-day mail order supplies. Call the customer service number on the coupon for help on how it can be used at mail order.
- Some private, commercial insurance companies will not allow their members to use coupon cards. One insurance company my pharmacy deals with bans their use. Some customers have called the insurance company directly, requesting they be allowed to use a coupon. The insurance company will sometimes give an approval.
- Not all pharmacies will take coupons. Call first to see if your pharmacy does. If they don't, call around.

Where Do I Get Coupons?

From your doctor. Many customers tell me that's where they obtained them. If your doctor doesn't have the coupon you need, look for it in pages 42-57. I've listed the drugs in alphabetical order to make it easy for you to find the ones you take. If you don't find one listed, skip to the information at the end of this chapter. In chapter 9 I'll give you other options for locating coupons, obtaining financial assistance from the drug companies, or from non-profit websites.

I realize not everyone reading this book has internet access. So as much as possible, I've included phone numbers to call for coupons and other types of financial help.

Before you attempt to use a coupon, I strongly recommend you read the fine print. I'm not kidding when I say you may need a magnifier to read what's on the coupon. Please read the information about how much the coupon will truly pay, whether or not it can be used with insurance, who's eligible, the number of times you can use the coupon, when it expires, and if it can be used at a mail order pharmacy.

Here's an example of why you need to read the fine print. The Lipitor co-pay card clearly says $4.00* Co-pay Card. That asterisk is a big clue. Here is how that $4.00 cost is explained at www.lipitor.com.

"To qualify for this offer, your out-of-pocket expense must be greater than $4 per prescription. If your out-of-pocket expenses for a 1-month supply (30 tablets) are $79 or less, you will pay $4 for a 1-month supply. If your out-of-pocket expenses for a 1-month supply (30 tablets) exceed $79, you qualify for up to $75 in savings for a 1-month supply. In either case, you can only qualify for up to $1,000 of savings per calendar year. After maximum of $1,000, you will pay usual monthly out-of-pocket costs."

I'll clarify it for you. You take the card to a local pharmacy to get a one month supply of Lipitor. To keep the math simple, let's say that one month of Lipitor costs $100.00.

You pay the $4.00
Manufacturer pays $75.00.
That leaves another $21.00 that *you* pay.
So in reality, you are paying $4.00 + $21.00 = $25.00

If you have insurance, the numbers will be different, depending on how much your insurance pays.

When Lipitor went generic in late 2011, I can't begin to count how many customers called to give me that coupon card, saying "The card says I'll only pay $4.00 for a 30-day supply so I should get a 90-day supply for $12.00". Nope. That's why you see asterisks on coupons. The asterisk is usually after the dollar amount. Nevertheless, there IS a savings.

Abilify

www.abilify.com

30-day free trial, plus continued savings tools and resources

Bristol-Myers Squibb   1-800-237-0051

Aciphex

www.aciphex.com

14 day free trial and monthly savings card

Janssen Pharmaceuticals   1-888-274-2378

Actoplus Met

www.actos.com

Click on "Special Savings Offers"

Takeda   1-888-838-9866

Adcirca

www.adcirca.com

Click the "Patient Assistance" tab

Eli Lilly and Company   1-877-864-8437

Aggrenox

www.aggrenox.com

Co-pay card

Boehringer Ingelheim Pharmaceuticals   1-855-277-2335

Alphagan

www.alphaganp.com/Patient/Default.aspx

Rebate

Allergan, Inc.   1-800-433-8871

Alvesco

www.alvesco.us

Instant rebate program

Sunovion Pharmaceuticals Inc.   1-888-394-7377

Ampyra

www.ampyra.com

Click on "Free 60 Day Trial of Ampyra"

Acordia Therapeutics, Inc.   1-888-881-1918

Androgel

www.androgeloffer.com

Coupon card

Abbott Laboratories   1-847-937-6100

Atacand

www.atacand.com

Coupon

AstraZeneca   1-800-236-9933

Avodart

www.avodart.com

Savings Card

Glaxo Smith Kline   1-888-825-5249

Avonex

www.avonex.com

30-day free trial

Biogen Idec   1-800-456-2255

Azor

www.azor.com

On the left side of the screen, click "Save on Co-pays"

Cards for 30 and 90-day supplies

Daiichi Sankyo, Inc   1-877-437-7763

Benefix

www.benefix.com

30-day free trial and a "Factor" savings card

Pfizer   1-888-240-9040

Betaseron

www.betaseron.com/betaplus/affordability

Zero Co-pay if you qualify

Bayer   1-800-788-1467

Celebrex

www.celebrex.com

Savings Card

Pfizer   1-888-678-2692

Cerezyme

www.cerezyme.com

Click the "Patients and Family" tab, and then scroll down to see the co-pay assistance link

Program runs through December 2012

Sanofi   1-800-745-4447

Chantix

www.chantix.com

Savings card

Pfizer   1-877-242-6849

Cialis

www.cialis.com

30-day free trial

Eli Lilly   1-800-545-5979

Cimzia

www.cimzia.com

Co-pay savings card

UCB Group of Companies   1-866-424-6942

Copaxone

www.sharedsolutions.com

Co-pay Solutions Card

Teva   1-800-887-8100

Crestor

www.crestor.com

Savings Card

AstraZeneca   1-888-729-4100

Cymbalta

www.cymbalta.com

30-day free trial

Eli Lilly   1-800-545-5979

Dexilant

www.dexilant.com

Click on "instant savings" on the menu options on the left side of the home page
Takeda   1-877-612-1146 (to get the card keep ignoring the system prompt about entering your Dexilant card number, eventually you will be transferred to a live representative)

Diovan

www.diovan.com
Coupon
Novartis   1-877-699-9975

Enbrel

www.enbrel.com
Enbrel support card
Amgen   1-888-436-2735

Estring

www.estring.com
Savings card
Pfizer   1-800-631-1181

Exelon Patch

www.exelonpatch.com
30-day free trial
Novartis   1-888-669-6682

Exforge

www.exforge.com

Coupon

Novartis   1-877-699-9975

Focalin XR

www.focalinxr.com

Savings card

Novartis   1-877-699-9975

Humira

www.humira.com/global/financial-assistance.aspx

Humira Protection Plan

Abbott Laboratories   1-800-448-6472

Intuniv

www.intuniv.com

Click on "Savings and Support"

Shire   1-800-828-2088

Januvia

www.januvia.com

30-day free trial and coupon card

Hover your mouse over the "Support For Type 2 Diabetes" tab, then choose "Special Offers"

Merck   1-800-444-2080

Kaletra

www.kaletra.com

Co-pay saving card

Click patient support tab, then click the co-pay savings card link in the middle of the page

Abbottt Laboratories   1- 888-525-3872

Kuvan

www.kuvan.com

30-day free trial

BioMarin Pharmaceutical Inc   1-866-906-6100

Lialda

www.lialda.com

Coupon

Shire Inc.   1-800-828-2088

Lipitor

https://www.lipitor.com/patients/lipitorforyou.aspx

Co-pay card − can be used with or without insurance

Pfizer   1-877-343-1239

Loestrin24 Fe7

www.loestrin24.com

Coupon

Warner Chilcott   1-800-521-8813 option 1

Lumigan

www.lumigan.com

Coupon

Allergan, Inc.   1-800-433-8871

Lunesta

www.lunesta.com

Coupon

Sunovion Pharmaceuticals Inc.   1-888-394-7377

Maxalt

www.maxalt.com

Free trial and a coupon

Merck   1-800-444-2080

Micardis

https://us.micardis.com/

30-day free trial

Boehringer Ingelheim Pharmaceuticals   1-800-243-0127

Nasonex

www.nasonex.com

Coupon

Merck   1-800-444-2080

Neulasta

www.neulasta.com

Coupon

Click on "Support Center", and then click "Neulasta Financial Help"

Amgen   1-805-447-1000

Nexium

www.pruplepill.com

Coupon

AstraZeneca   1-800-236-9933

Niaspan

www.niaspan.com

Heart Alliance Program

Abbott Laboratories   1-847-937-6100

NuvaRing

www.nuvaring.com

Click "Savings and Support" on the left side of the screen

Call McKesson Corporation   1-877-264-2440

Omnaris

www.omnaris.com

Coupon

Sunovion Pharmaceuticals Inc.   1-888-394-7377

Opana ER

www.opana.com

Coupon

Endo Pharmaceuticals   1-800-462-3636

Oracea

www.oracea.com

Coupon

Galderma Laboratories   1-866-735-4137

Orencia

www.orencia.com

Coupon

Bristol-Myers Squibb   1-800-673-6242

Ortho Tri-Cyclen Lo

www.thepill.com

Coupon

Janssen Pharmaceuticals   1-800-526-7736

Pataday

www.pataday.com

Rebate

Norvartis   1-800-862-5266

Patanol

www.patanol.com

Rebate

Norvartis   1-800-862-5266

Pulmozyme

www.pulmozyme.com

Co-pay card

Genentech   1-800-690-3023

Rapamune

www.rapamune.com

Co-pay card

Pfizer   1-800-879-3477

Relpax

www.relpax.com

Coupon

Pfizer   1-800-926-5334

Remicade

www.remistart.com

Rebate Program

Contact AccessOne at 1-888-222-3771

Renvela

www.renvalue.com

Co-pay card for those with AND without insurance

Call Renassist at 1-800-847-0069

Reyataz

www.ReyatazSavings.com

Savings card − first use must take place by December 31, 2012

Bristol-Myers Squibb   1-888-281-8981

Rilutek

www.rilutek.com

Savings card

Sanofi   1-800-745-8835

Rituxan

www.rituxan.com/hem/co-pay/index.html

Bioncology copay card

Genentech   1-888-249-4918

Sensipar

www.SensiparPharmacyCard.com

Sensipar Pharmacy Card

Amgen   1-866-711-4162

Simponi

www.simponi.com

Click "Get Your Support Your Way", then click on" Medication Cost Support"

Janssen Biotech   1-877-697-4676

Solodyn ER

www.solodyn.com

Savings card

Medicis   1-800-550-5115

Spectracef

www.spectracef.com

Coupon

Cornerstone Therapeutics   1-888-661-9260

Spiriva

www.spiriva.com

Click on "Patient Support"

Boehringer Ingelheim Pharmaceuticals   1-800-243-0127

Stalera

www.stelarainfo.com/patient-support

Savings card

Janssen Biotech   1-877-783-5272

Strattera

www.strattera.com

30-day free trial for adults, children and teens

Lilly   1-800-545-5979

Sustiva

www.bmscopayprogramsusrey.com/bmscopayprogramsusrey/index.html

Coupon

Bristol-Myers Squibb   1-888-281-8981

Symbicort

www.mysymbicort.com

First fill is free

AstraZeneca   1-877-916-4312

Tasigna

www.tasigna.com

Co-pay program

Novartis   1-866-972-8313

Tazoarc Gel

www.tazorac.com

Rebate

Novartis   1-800-245-5356

TOBI

www.tobitime.com

Coupon – click on "TOBI Care"

Novartis   1-877-999-8624

Travatan and Travatan Z

www.travatanz.com

Savings Card – for those beginning treatment and those continuing treatment

Alcon   1-800-862-5266

Trilipix

www.trilipx.com

Trilipix Care Program - Scroll down on the home page and click on "Save Now"

Abbott Laboratories   1-847-937-6100

Truvada

www.truvada.com

Co-pay card

Gilead Science, Inc.   1-888-358-0398

Uribel

www.uribelinfo.com

Coupon card

Mission Pharmaceutical   1-210-696-8400

Valcyte

www.valcyte.com

Co-pay card

Genentech   1-877-698-2549

Velcade

www.velcade.com

Click on "Paying For Treatment"

Millennium Pharmaceuticals   1-866-835-2233, option 2

Vesicare

www.vesicare.com

Free trial and a coupon – Click on "Savings and Resources"

Astellas Pharma, Inc.   1-800-888-7704

Victoza

www.victoza.com

Click on "Save on Victoza prescriptions

Novo Nordisk   1-877-905-1126

Viread

www.viread.com/en/my_access.aspx

Coupon card

Gilead Science, Inc.   1-877-627-0415

Vivelle-DOT

www.vivelledot.com

Free trial and you can request a free non-medicated sample

Novogyne Pharmaceuticals   1-888-669-6682

Vytorin

www.vytorin.com

Free trial and a coupon

Merck - financial help phone number   1-800-727-5400

Vyvanse

www.vyvanse.com

Savings card

Shire   1-800-828-2088

Welchol

www.welchol.com

Savings card

Daiichi Sankyo   1-866-747-1357

Xeloda

www.xeloda.com

Co-pay card

Genentech   1-855-692-6729

Xolair

www.xolair.com

Co-pay card - Click on "Financial Resources for Xolair Patients"

Genentech   1-877-411-8641

Zetia

www.zetia.com

Free trial and coupon − on the left side of screen click "Special Offers for Zetia"

Merck - financial help phone number   1-800-727-5400

Zetonna

www.zetonna.com

Coupon

Sunovion Pharmaceuticals Inc.   1-888-394-7377

Zytiga

www.zytiga.com

ZytigaOne™ Support Instant Savings Program

Janssen   1-855-998-4421

I used the list of brand name drugs in chapter two when searching for coupons. This list is by no means a complete list of all coupons for brand names. It's a list of all that I could find for brand drugs that have yet to go generic.

More co-pay coupons for brand names can be found at

www.internetdrugcoupons.com.

If you have no insurance, you can still use the search function at this site to find coupons that are meant to be used without insurance.

State Help

Help For the Uninsured, Low Income, and in Some Cases, the Insured

Help from states is a mixed bag. Some are discount cards that everyone in the state can get, regardless of income or age. Those cards are generally meant to be used by the uninsured. But those who have insurance can use the cards to bring down the cost of medications their insurance doesn't cover.

Other states only offer help to people over 65 and those with disabilities. Some states only offer help to those at the poverty level.

Unfortunately, many states offer no help at all. Below is a list of the states that give help in one form or another. I've listed them in alphabetical order.

ALABAMA

www.alabamaageline.gov/seniorx.cfm

1-800-243-5463

SenioRx/Wellness program for Alabamans 55 or older.

ARIZONA

azgovernor.gov/coppercard

1-888-227-8315

- Every Arizonan is entitled to a free CoppeRX Card.
- All commonly prescribed medications are included in the program.
- Present your card at any of the more than 1,000 participating pharmacies throughout Arizona.
- Save an average of 20% off the regular retail price.

You can print your card at this site.

ARKANSAS

Arkansas Health Care Access Foundation, Inc.

www.ahcaf.org

1-800-950-8233 or 1-501-221-3033

Email: info@ahcaf.org

CALIFORNIA

Drug discount program for Medicare recipients

www.dhcs.ca.gov/individuals/Pages/PresDrgDisPrgmMedRcpts.Aspx

1-800-434-0222

Show your Medicare card at participating pharmacies to get drugs at Medi-Cal prices (when paying out of pocket).

CONNECTICUT

www.connpace.com

1-800-423-5026 or 860-269-2029 in the Hartford area

ConnPACE is a service that helps eligible senior citizens and people with disabilities afford the cost of most prescription medicines as well as insulin and insulin syringes.

You may qualify for ConnPACE if:

- You are age 65 or older.
- You are 18 or older and have a disability.
- You are NOT eligible for Medicare.

DELAWARE

Prescription Assistance Program

www.dhss.delaware.gov/dhss/dmma/dpap.html

1-800-996-9969

You must be 65 or over.

The goal of the Delaware Prescription Assistance Program (DPAP) is to help pay for prescription medications for elderly and/or disabled individuals who cannot afford the full cost of their prescriptions. The program is designed to aid eligible individuals who have no prescription insurance other than Medicare Part D, and whose income is at or below 200% of the Federal Poverty Level (FPL), or whose prescription costs exceed 40% of their income.

FLORIDA

www.floridadiscountdrugcard.com

Enroll online, or call: 1-866-341-8894

TTY Users may call: 1-866-763-9630

All Floridians can sign up for the Florida Discount Drug Card to save on their prescription medications. Use this website to print a card, locate a pharmacy, and compare prescription drug prices.

HAWAII

Hawaii State Pharmacy Assistance Program (Hawaii SPAP)

www.med-quest.us/eligibility/EligPrograms.html

1-866-878-9769

Assistance listed for various segments of Hawaii's population.

ILLINOIS

www.illinoisrxbuyingclub.com

1-866-215-3463   (TTY) 1-866-215-3479

- Discounts on prescription drugs, both brand name and generic.
- Savings average 20%; individual discounts may vary.
- The card is accepted at 50,000 locations nationwide. There are 2,500 pharmacies in Illinois, customers can go anywhere in the U.S.
- There are income limits.
- There is a $10.00 non-refundable, annual administrative fee.

KENTUCKY

www.healthkentucky.org

For very low income only

1-502-564-8966 extension 4216

LOUISIANA

www.louisianaseniorx.org

1-877-340-9100

Senior help only

MAINE – for the elderly

www.maine.gov/dhhs/oads/aging/resource/lc_drugs.htm

1-866-796-2463   TTY: Maine relay 711

- 80% minus $2.00 of the cost of all generic prescription drugs on the Preferred Drug List.

- 80% minus $2.00 of the cost of brand-name medications on the Preferred Drug List for the treatment of diabetes, heart disease, high blood pressure, chronic lung disease (emphysema and asthma), arthritis, anticoagulation, Hyperlipidemia (high cholesterol), incontinence, thyroid disease, osteoporosis, (bone density loss,), Parkinson's Disease, glaucoma, Multiple Sclerosis, and ALS (Lou Gehrig's Disease).

MAINE – non-seniors

www.maine.gov/dhhs/mainerx

1-866-796-2463   TTY / TDD 1-800-423-4331

Discount card

Qualification based on monthly gross income.

MARYLAND

www.medbankmd.org

1-877-435-7755

Click "Discount Card" on the left hand side of the page.

Call Medbank to see if you are eligible for a free prescription program.

MARYLAND – Medicare Assistance

www.marylandspdap.com

1-800-551-5995   TTY/TDD - 1-800-877-5156

To participate in the Senior Prescription Drug Assistance Program, individuals must meet the following eligibility requirements:

- Show residency in Maryland for at least six months.
- Be a Medicare recipient.
- Have an income at or below 300% of the Federal Poverty Level.

MASSACHUSETTS

www.massresources.org/prescription-advantage.html

1-800-243-4636   TTY: 1-877-610-0241

Prescription Advantage is a state-sponsored prescription drug insurance plan for Massachusetts seniors and disabled residents. For people on Medicare, Prescription Advantage helps pay Part D Prescription Drug Plan costs. For people not on Medicare, the program provides primary prescription drug coverage.

Another program

MassMedLine

1-866-633-1617

Its staff of trained clinical pharmacists and case managers will explore all possible ways to reduce your costs while encouraging safe medication use and good health practices. They work closely with you and your physician to ensure the best care.

MICHIGAN

www.mihealth.org/mirx/index.html

Application request, enrollment questions, or lost cards:

1-866-755-6479 (Press 2, then 1)

This is a prescription drug discount program for Michigan residents who do not have any prescription drug coverage.

MINNESOTA

http://www.mnaging.org/advisor/SLL.htm

1-800-333-2433

RxConnect is a state sponsored, objective, neutral service managed by the Minnesota Board on Aging's Senior LinkAges Line. Even though the Senior LinkAge Line staff answers the phones, the service isn't limited to people who are seniors. Staff are trained and certified as Health Insurance Counselors and have a special expertise in helping people with prescription drug costs.

People of all ages who need assistance in finding help with their prescription drug costs can call RxConnect. The staff will discuss all pharmaceutical options with callers. Depending on the options available, appropriate and chosen by the caller, RxConnect can help complete the paperwork and prepare the information for mailing. Help is available on a one-to-one basis, over the phone or in person.

MISSOURI

www.morx.mo.gov/#

1-800-375-1406

You may be eligible if you are:

- A resident of the State of Missouri. **and**
- Enrolled in a Medicare Part D Plan.
- Single — with an annual gross household income of $21,660 or less or.
- Married — with an annual gross household income of $29,140 or less.

MONTANA

www.dphhs.mt.gov/prescriptiondrug/bigsky.shtml

Apply online or call: 1-866-369-1233

Eligibility Criteria:

- Montana is your primary state of residence.
- Must be a Medicare recipient.
- Must meet generous income criteria.
- Income less than $22,340 (single person) or $30,260 (two person household).

NEVADA – Senior RX

www.dhhs.nv.gov/SeniorRx.htm

1-866-303-6323 Option 7

For those who are Not Medicare Eligible:

- No monthly premium.
- No deductible.
- Co-payments of $10 for generics or $25 for preferred brands.
- Annual coverage limit of $5,100.

For those who are Medicare Eligible:

- Help with monthly premiums for Medicare Part D Prescription Drug Plan (if not qualified for maximum help from Medicare with that expense).
- Help with prescription costs after reaching the Medicare Part D coverage limit.

NEVADA – Disability RX

www.dhhs.nv.gov/DisabilityRx.htm

1-866-303-6323

Eligibility requirements:

- Age 18 through 61 with verifiable disability.
- Nevada resident continuously for at least the last 12 months.
- Annual income no more than $26,836 for singles and $35,773 for couples.

NEW HAMPSHIRE

www.healthynh.com/fhc/initiatives/access/medicationbridge.php

1-603-225-0900

Click on "List of N.H. Medication Bridge Program Sites" to see the list of facilities that provide help.

NEW JERSEY

Help for the Aged and Disabled

www.nj.gov/health/seniorbenefits/paaddetail.shtml

Call toll free Hotline 1-800-792-9745

New Jersey Prescription Drug Price Registry

www6.state.nj.us/LPSCA_DRUG/index.jsp

This site helps consumers compare the retail prices charged by many pharmacies for the 150 most-frequently prescribed prescription drugs.

By comparing prices here, consumers can see what a pharmacy has reported to the State that it charged for a specific prescription drug. Comparing the prices listed in this registry will help a consumer find the pharmacy in his or her area with the lowest retail price for a specific prescription drug.

NEW MEXICO

Discount Prescription Drug Program (DPDP).

www.nmrhca.state.nm.us/Home/DPDP/Details.aspx

1-800-233-2576

The DPDP is available to all residents of New Mexico regardless of age, whether or not you have other insurance. If you have other insurance, you cannot use both cards for the same drug purchase; you can use whichever one benefits you the most for that purchase.

NEW YORK

Elderly Pharmaceutical Insurance Coverage (EPIC) Program

www.health.ny.gov/health_care/epic\

Apply online, or call 1-800-332-3742   TTY 1-800-290-9138

To join EPIC, a senior must:

- be a New York State resident age 65 or older.
- have an annual income below $35,000 if single or $50,000 if married.
- be enrolled or eligible to be enrolled in a Medicare Part D plan (no exceptions). and
- not be receiving full Medicaid benefits.

NORTH CAROLINA

Help for low-income seniors

www.healthwellnc.com/NCRx.aspx

1-919-981-5000

NCRx is a prescription drug assistance plan to help low-income seniors participate in the federal Medicare Part D prescription drug program. NCRx is available to low-income seniors who meet the eligibility requirements. The program pays up to $29 toward monthly premiums for Medicare Prescription Drug Plans that work with NCRx.

NORTH DAKOTA

www.nd.gov/ndins/prescription

No financial help from the state.

If you call 1-888-575-6611, you will get help finding a patient assistance program with a drug manufacturer. Or simply read the next chapter of this book.

OHIO

Ohio's Best Rx

www.ohiobestrx.org/en/index.aspx

Sign up online or call 1-866-923-7879

TTY Users may dial 711 for Relay Service.

Ohio's Best Rx Card is available to all Ohio residents without restriction and is accepted at over 60,000 pharmacies nationwide. Ohio residents who qualify based on age or income status are eligible to receive additional savings.

Use the website to print a card, locate a pharmacy, and compare prescription drug prices.

OKLAHOMA

Rx for Oklahoma

okcommerce.gov/community-resources/grants-and-funding-programs/rx-for-oklahoma/

1-877-794-6552

No financial help from the state. They will take your information, find the right patient assistance program for you, and help you with the paperwork. Since the process can take 30-days, this only applies to maintenance medications.

OREGON

Oregon Prescription Drug Plan

www.oregon.gov/OHA/pharmacy/OPDP/index.shtml

Enroll online or call 1-800-913-4146

- Free enrollment.
- All Oregonians are eligible.
- Average savings of 50% on prescriptions. Highest discount is on generics.
- There is no paperwork required and no age or income limit.

The card is meant to be used by those with no insurance. People with insurance can use the card to purchase medications not covered by their insurance.

Click "Look up Drug Cost" on the left hand side of the page, to price your drug for both a 30-day and 90-day supply.

Other Oregon help

http://cms.oregon.gov/oha/pharmacy/Pages/careassist/index.aspx

CAREassist helps people living with HIV or AIDS pay for medical care expenses

1-971-673-0144 or 1-800-805-2313

PENNSYLVANIA

www.portal.state.pa.us/portal/server.pt/community/prescription
_assistance/17942

1-800-225-7223

PACE, PACENET, and PACE plus Medicare are Pennsylvania's prescription assistance programs for older adults, offering low-cost prescription medication to qualified residents, age 65 and older.

Income levels apply.

This website contains a pricing tool and links for prescription help for people with HIV/AIDS and other diseases.

You can call the Patient Assistant Program Clearing House at 1-800-955-0989 for assistance in finding a patient assistance program that's right for you.

RHODE ISLAND

Rhode Island Pharmaceutical Assistance to the Elderly (ripae)

www.dea.ri.gov/programs/prescription_assist.php

1-401-462-3000   TTY 1-401-462-0740

Rhode Island residents 65 or older, who meet specific income guidelines, are eligible to enroll in RIPAE. RIPAE members are mandated to have enrollment in a Medicare Part D plan. Member co-payments for prescriptions used to treat medical conditions listed in Category A are based on a sliding scale. RIPAE members 65 and older can purchase medications listed in Category B at the discounted RIPAE price.

Income levels apply.

TENNESSEE
www.covertennessee.gov/web/cover_rx.html
Program is administered by Express Scripts   1-888-560-2649

Applicants must meet the following eligibility guidelines:
* Tennessee resident (six months).
* Age 19-64.
* U.S. citizen or qualified legal alien.
* Household income at or below 250% federal poverty level (FPL).
* Cannot have pharmacy coverage such as TennCare or employer insurance.
* Cannot have Medicare (any part including A, B, C or D).
* CoverRx members may participate in other discount drug programs, such as those offered by retail stores.

At the website you can look up the drug formulary and see pricing.

VERMONT
Vermont State Pharmacy Assistant Plans
www.q1medicare.com/PartDSPAPVermontVPharmVHAPPharVSCRIPT.php
1-800-250-8427
For those over 65 or disabled who are on Social Security.
Income limits apply.

WASHINGTON
Washington Prescription Drug Plan

www.rx.wa.gov

Enroll online or call 1-800-913-4146   Customer service is 1-800-913-4311

Who is eligible to join WPDP?

- Washington State residents.
- No age or income restrictions.
- Each person must enroll individually.

Who can benefit from the WPDP discount card?

- Washington State residents.
- People who have a high-deductible health plan such as a Health Savings Account (HSA) may be able to use the WPDP discount card when paying down the deductible (check with your HSA plan for details).
- People who have no insurance coverage.
- People who have medical coverage but no prescription drug benefit.
- People who have prescription drug coverage through their employer, but it does not cover the drug they need.

How much does it cost?
- The WPDP is FREE.
- No annual fee and no hidden costs.

Click "Drug Prices" in the yellow box on the home page to price your medications.

WISCONSIN

Badger Rx Gold

www.badgerrxgold.com/badgerrxgold/default.asp

1-866-809-9382

BadgerRx Gold is a prescription drug program that makes prescription medications accessible and affordable to people in Wisconsin who are uninsured or underinsured.

You pay a yearly, non-refundable fee. Before you enroll, call first to see what your savings will be.

WYOMING

www.health.wyo.gov/healthcarefin/pharmacy/PDAP.html

1-800-438-5785

The program is for those at the poverty level.

9

Patient Assistance Programs, Low-Income Clinics, and Coupons for the Uninsured

If you have no insurance and/or are classified as low income, there are many places to get help. For those whose incomes are low enough, your best option on high-cost drugs is to contact the manufacturers of those drugs to get your medication at little or no cost, through a Patient Assistance Program (PAP).

The best place by far to find those programs is:

www.pparx.org   1-888-477-2669

This site contains a treasure-trove of information.

You can find help with:
- Medicare D
- Medicare/CHIP programs
- Patient Assistance Programs – covers more than just getting help with the cost of meds
- Co-payment programs
- Free low-cost clinic finder
- Savings cards
- Additional resources

Since there is far more information at that website than I can put into this book, I recommend you visit their site. If you don't have internet access, call them and they'll gladly help you.

Before applying for assistance directly from a pharmaceutical manufacturer, you need to know which one to contact. The label on your medication bottle will tell you. The drug company's name will be after the word Manufacturer or the abbreviation MFG. If the label was on a box that you threw out, or is unreadable, call the pharmacy that filled it and ask a pharmacist who makes that drug.

No Insurance? Coupons You Can Use

Since most manufacturer coupons can only be used with insurance, people with no insurance need to look elsewhere. Fortunately, there are many coupons you can use. They are all over the internet so you will need access to the web to get these coupons. I've listed one site that has a phone number for those of you who don't have a computer. Unlike manufacturer coupons, which will show a specific dollar amount that you'll save, these coupons will say "save up to 75% off" or similar numbers. Note the "up to" part.

At **www.internetdrugcoupons.com** you'll find a huge number of coupons. This site has no phone number for you to call, so if you don't have internet access, try the site listed below. I've called their customer service number and found them helpful and willing to answer all my questions.

Help Rx
http://www.helprx.info   1-800-776-1760

Their customer service representatives can send you coupons and/or an Rx card. Check their FAQ section to see how the coupons work and how to obtain one if you don't have a printer.

Another useful website for locating PAP's, coupons and Medicare D information is: **www.rxassist.org.**

They have no phone number but can be contacted through e-mail.

For those with rare disorders:

www.rarediseases.org

1-203-744-0100

Voicemail only   1-800-999-6673

10

More Savings

Call Around

First, see if the generics you take are available at pharmacies offering $4.00 for a 30-day supply and $10.00 for a 90-day supply. If some aren't, then call around to as many pharmacies in your area as possible for cash prices. Prices will vary from pharmacy to pharmacy. Some of those pharmacies might offer a cash incentive to move your prescriptions to them, so take that into account when calling. If the pharmacy you frequent doesn't have the lowest price, ask if they will match the lowest price you found.

Veterans Administration

For part of 2004, I was between jobs and had no medical or prescription insurance. During that period, I had the misfortune of having a sinus infection spread to my eyes. On the upside, I'm an Army veteran and was registered with the local VA hospital. I headed to the emergency room – twice. The first visit cost me a grand total of $7.00, for the eye drops I was prescribed. I was told if that medication didn't work within a few days to come back for further help. I had to go back and was rushed up to the eye clinic. Again, I paid $7.00 for another prescription for eye drops. The ophthalmologist had me return for follow up visits. None of those visits cost me a cent.

Depending on which priority group you are placed in, your cost is now either $8.00 or $9.00 for non-service connected conditions. Great prices if you are an eligible veteran.

www.va.gov/healthbenefits/online

Click on FAQ and search with "prescriptions" to learn more.

Over The Counter (OTC) Drugs

Once in a while, a medications' status will change from requiring a prescription to becoming available without a prescription. This results in a saving if you had no insurance when you purchased the prescription medication. For those who purchased the prescription medication through insurance, you probably will find that you are paying more for the OTC medication.

Here's an example explaining why. Not long ago, fexofenadine − the generic of Allegra − became an OTC. When that happened, insurance companies stopped covering it. So that lovely, low $10 co-pay you had for a 90-day supply disappeared. You now had to purchase it at a local pharmacy for roughly $17 dollars for a 30-day supply.

To keep OTC costs down:

- Pay attention to the ads in your mailbox.
- Look for in-store specials.
- Look for a store brand version − it will cost less.

Pick up your phone, get online, and start saving now!

INDEX